Atkins Diet Simple Guide for Beginners

Understanding the Benefits of Atkins Diet

By

Glyn Hubert

Table of Contents

CHAPTER 1

Introduction

The Atkins Diet is a well-known and widely practiced low-carbohydrate diet that has gained immense popularity over the years for its potential to help individuals shed excess weight and improve their overall health. This section will provide a comprehensive overview of the Atkins Diet, delving into what it is, its associated benefits, and addressing common misconceptions.

1.1 What is the Atkins Diet?

The Atkins Diet, developed by Dr. Robert C. Atkins in the early 1970s, is a dietary regimen that primarily focuses on reducing carbohydrate intake while emphasizing the consumption of proteins and fats. It operates on the fundamental premise that limiting carbohydrates forces the body to enter a state of ketosis, where it burns fat for energy instead of carbohydrates. The diet is structured into four distinct phases:

- **Induction Phase:** This initial phase severely restricts carbohydrate intake, typically to under 20-25 grams per day. During this phase, the body shifts into ketosis, jump-starting fat burning.

- **Balancing Phase:** In this phase, carbohydrate intake is gradually increased while closely monitoring the body's response to carbohydrates. The goal is to determine the individual's carbohydrate tolerance while continuing to lose weight.

- **Pre-Maintenance Phase:** Here, the carbohydrate intake increases further, but at a slower pace. This phase helps prepare individuals for long-term weight maintenance.

- **Maintenance Phase:** The final phase allows for a higher carbohydrate intake, but it's still lower than the typical Western diet. The focus is on maintaining weight while enjoying a balanced diet.

One of the distinguishing features of the Atkins Diet is that it does not restrict calorie consumption but rather the source of those calories. By limiting carbohydrates, the diet aims to regulate blood sugar levels, reduce insulin spikes, and ultimately promote fat loss.

1.2 Benefits of the Atkins Diet

The Atkins Diet has garnered attention for several potential benefits:

- **Weight Loss:** Many individuals have reported significant weight loss while following the Atkins Diet, particularly during the initial phases when carbohydrate intake is restricted. The shift to fat burning can lead to rapid fat loss.

- **Improved Blood Sugar Control:** By reducing carbohydrate intake, the diet can help stabilize blood sugar levels, making it particularly beneficial for individuals with type 2 diabetes or those at risk of developing it.

- **Reduced Triglycerides:** Lower carbohydrate consumption can lead to decreased triglyceride levels, which is a positive marker for heart health.

- **Increased HDL Cholesterol:** Some people experience an increase in high-density lipoprotein (HDL) cholesterol, which is considered "good" cholesterol and can contribute to better cardiovascular health.

- **Appetite Control:** Protein and fat are more satiating than carbohydrates, which can help control appetite and reduce overeating.

- **Improved Energy Levels:** Many followers of the Atkins Diet report increased energy levels and improved mental clarity.

- **Flexible Food Choices:** The diet allows for a variety of food choices, making it adaptable to individual preferences and dietary restrictions.

1.3 Common Misconceptions

Despite its popularity and potential benefits, the Atkins Diet has also faced its fair share of misconceptions and criticisms:

- **Unlimited Fat Consumption:** One common misconception is that the Atkins Diet encourages unlimited consumption of high-fat foods. While fat intake is encouraged, it should come from healthy sources like avocados, nuts, and olive oil.

- **Lack of Nutritional Balance:** Critics argue that the diet may lack nutritional balance because of its strict carbohydrate restriction, potentially leading to deficiencies in essential nutrients.

- **Unsustainability:** Some individuals believe that the Atkins Diet is unsustainable in the long term due to its carbohydrate restrictions. However, the diet does have phases aimed at transitioning to a more balanced and sustainable eating pattern.

- **All Carbohydrates are Equal:** The Atkins Diet emphasizes differentiating between "good" and "bad" carbohydrates. It encourages the consumption of fiber-rich, nutrient-dense carbohydrates and discourages refined sugars and highly processed foods.

- **Health Concerns:** Some have expressed concerns about the diet's impact on kidney function and cholesterol levels. It's

essential to consult with a
healthcare professional before
starting any diet plan,
especially if you have
preexisting health conditions.

The Atkins Diet is a low-carbohydrate dietary approach that has been lauded for its potential to promote weight loss and improve various aspects of metabolic health. However, it is not without its controversies and misconceptions. As with any diet, it's crucial to approach it with an understanding of its principles, individualize it to your needs, and seek professional guidance when necessary to ensure it aligns with your health goals and overall well-being.

CHAPTER 2

Understanding the Atkins Diet

To fully grasp the Atkins Diet and how it operates, it is essential to delve into its structure, which is divided into distinct phases. These phases are designed to guide individuals through a gradual transformation of their eating habits while achieving specific health and weight loss goals. In this section, we will explore the four key phases of the Atkins Diet.

2.1 Phases of the Atkins Diet

The Atkins Diet is divided into four sequential phases, each serving a unique purpose and allowing individuals to progressively adapt to a lower carbohydrate intake while achieving their desired health outcomes. These phases are as follows:

2.1.1 Induction Phase

- *Duration and Goals*: The Induction Phase marks the beginning of the Atkins Diet and typically lasts for about two weeks. The primary goal during this phase is to induce a state of ketosis, where the body shifts from using carbohydrates as its primary energy source to burning stored fat.

- *Allowed Foods*: Individuals in the Induction Phase are encouraged to consume foods that are high in healthy fats, moderate in protein, and very low in carbohydrates. Examples include meat, poultry, fish, eggs, butter, oils, and select low-carb vegetables like spinach and broccoli.

- *Sample Meal Plan*: A typical day in the Induction Phase might include meals such as scrambled eggs with spinach and bacon for breakfast, a salad with grilled chicken for lunch, and salmon with steamed broccoli for dinner.

- *Tips for Success*: Staying hydrated, incorporating adequate electrolytes, and monitoring carbohydrate intake closely are vital for success during this phase. It's also essential to read food labels carefully to identify hidden sugars and carbohydrates.

2.1.2 Balancing Phase

- *Transitioning to the Balancing Phase*: After completing the Induction Phase, individuals progress to the Balancing Phase. The duration of this phase varies depending on individual goals, but it typically involves gradually increasing carbohydrate intake.

- *Adjusting Carbohydrate Intake*: In the Balancing Phase, individuals experiment with different levels of carbohydrate consumption to identify their carbohydrate tolerance. They continue to lose weight but at a slower rate compared to the Induction Phase.

- *Sample Meal Plan*: During this phase, a meal plan might include a wider variety of low-carb vegetables, small servings of berries, and slightly larger portions of nuts and seeds. Whole grains may be reintroduced in moderation.

- *Staying on Track*: It's crucial to maintain a balance between carbohydrates and other nutrients during this phase. Tracking food intake and monitoring weight loss progress is essential to avoid overconsumption of carbohydrates.

2.1.3 Pre-Maintenance Phase

- *Preparing for Maintenance*: The Pre-Maintenance Phase acts as a bridge between active weight loss and long-term maintenance. The goal is to fine-tune eating habits and gradually transition to a sustainable carbohydrate intake.

- *Gradually Reintroducing Carbs*: Individuals slowly reintroduce more carbohydrates into their diet, such as fruits, legumes, and whole grains. This phase helps identify the maximum carbohydrate intake that allows weight maintenance.

- *Monitoring Your Progress*: Regularly assessing how different carbohydrate levels affect weight and energy levels is essential during the Pre-

Maintenance Phase. Adjustments are made as needed.

- *Sample Meal Plan*: A sample meal plan may include a wider variety of fruits, such as apples and berries, and slightly larger portions of complex carbohydrates like quinoa or sweet potatoes.

2.1.4 Maintenance Phase

- *Long-Term Sustainability*: The Maintenance Phase is where individuals have reached their desired weight and aim to maintain it. Carbohydrate intake is at its highest level during this phase but is still lower than that of the typical Western diet.

- *Finding Your Carb Tolerance*: By now, individuals have identified their carbohydrate tolerance, ensuring that they can maintain their weight without gaining it back.

- *Meal Planning for Maintenance*: The focus during this phase is on a balanced diet that includes carbohydrates, proteins, and fats. The emphasis is on choosing nutrient-dense, whole foods.

- *Avoiding Common Pitfalls*: Maintaining a healthy lifestyle, staying active, and avoiding a return to unhealthy eating habits are essential for long-term success during the Maintenance Phase.

Understanding these phases of the Atkins Diet is crucial for anyone considering or already following this dietary approach. It allows individuals to tailor their diet to their specific goals, whether it's rapid weight loss, better blood sugar control, or long-term weight maintenance. Moreover, it highlights the importance of continuous self-monitoring and adjustments to ensure that the diet aligns with individual health and wellness objectives.

2.2 How the Atkins Diet Works

The Atkins Diet operates on a unique principle of carbohydrate restriction to alter the body's metabolism and promote weight loss and improved health. Here's how the Atkins Diet works:

- **Carbohydrate Restriction**: The fundamental premise of the Atkins Diet is to significantly reduce carbohydrate intake. This reduction in carbs forces the body to find an alternative source of energy because it can no longer rely on glucose derived from carbohydrates.

- **Ketosis**: When carbohydrate intake is limited to a very low level, the body enters a metabolic state known as ketosis. In ketosis, the liver begins to convert stored fat into molecules called ketones, which are used as an energy source instead of glucose. This shift to burning fat for fuel can result in weight loss.

- **Stabilizing Blood Sugar**: By reducing carbohydrate intake, the Atkins Diet helps stabilize blood sugar levels. When you consume carbohydrates, they are broken down into glucose, causing blood sugar levels to rise. This can lead to insulin spikes and energy crashes. With fewer carbohydrates, blood sugar remains more stable, reducing hunger and cravings.

- **Promoting Fat Loss**: Ketosis promotes the breakdown of stored fat for energy, leading to fat loss. This is why many people experience rapid weight loss, particularly during the initial phases of the Atkins Diet.

- **Satiety**: Foods rich in protein and fat are more satiating than carbohydrates. This increased feeling of fullness can help control appetite and reduce overall calorie intake.

- **Customization**: The Atkins Diet is highly customizable. It offers four phases, each with different levels of carbohydrate intake, allowing individuals to tailor the diet to their specific goals, preferences, and health conditions.

2.3 Foods Allowed and Restricted

The Atkins Diet emphasizes specific categories of foods, both allowed and restricted, depending on the phase of the diet:

Foods Allowed:

1. **Protein**: Lean meats such as chicken, turkey, beef, pork, and fish are encouraged. Eggs are also a staple in the diet.

2. **Fats**: Healthy fats like avocados, nuts, seeds, olive oil, and coconut oil are permitted.

3. **Low-Carb Vegetables**: Non-starchy vegetables such as leafy greens, broccoli, cauliflower, and bell peppers are included in most phases.

4. **Dairy**: Some dairy products like cheese and full-fat yogurt can be consumed in moderation, primarily in later phases.

5. **Nuts and Seeds**: These provide healthy fats and can be eaten in moderation.

6. **Berries**: In moderation, low-carb fruits like strawberries, blueberries, and raspberries can be included in later phases.

7. **Sweeteners**: Some artificial sweeteners like stevia and erythritol are allowed for those with a sweet tooth.

Foods Restricted:

1. **High-Carb Foods**: Foods high in carbohydrates are restricted, including bread, pasta, rice, and sugary snacks.

2. **Sugars**: Added sugars, sweets, and sugary beverages are not allowed.

3. **Starchy Vegetables**: Starchy vegetables like potatoes and corn are limited or avoided in the early phases.

4. **Grains**: Grains, cereals, and most grain-based products are restricted.

5. **Fruits (initially)**: High-carb fruits like bananas, grapes, and oranges are limited in the early phases but can be reintroduced in moderation in later phases.

6. **Processed Foods**: Highly processed and packaged foods are discouraged due to their high carb content and additives.

It's important to note that while the Atkins Diet restricts carbohydrates, it does not impose strict calorie limits. Instead, it focuses on the source of calories, encouraging the consumption of nutrient-dense, whole foods. Additionally, the progression through the four phases of the diet allows for a gradual reintroduction of carbohydrates, making it more sustainable for long-term dietary habits. Individuals should consult with a healthcare professional before starting the Atkins Diet, especially if they have underlying health conditions or concerns about nutrient balance.

CHAPTER 3

Getting Started

Embarking on the Atkins Diet requires careful planning and preparation to ensure success. In this section, we will explore the crucial steps to take when getting started on the Atkins Diet, including setting clear goals and preparing your kitchen for the dietary changes ahead.

3.1 Setting Your Goals

Before diving into any diet, including the Atkins Diet, it's essential to define your specific goals. Your goals will shape your approach to the diet and help you stay motivated throughout the journey. Here are some common goals people have when starting the Atkins Diet:

- **Weight Loss**: Many individuals turn to the Atkins Diet with the primary goal of shedding excess pounds. Determine how much weight you aim to lose and set realistic, achievable milestones.

- **Blood Sugar Control**: If you have type 2 diabetes or are at risk for developing it, your goal may be to stabilize blood sugar levels and reduce the need for medication.

- **Improved Overall Health**: Some people are drawn to the Atkins Diet to improve their overall health, including reducing inflammation, lowering cholesterol levels, and boosting energy.

- **Better Eating Habits**: The Atkins Diet can help break unhealthy eating patterns and promote a more balanced diet.

- **Long-Term Weight Maintenance**: If you've already lost weight and want to maintain it, the Atkins Diet can serve as a tool for sustainable weight management.

Once you've established your goals, consider breaking them down into smaller, manageable objectives. This can make the journey feel less daunting and help you track your progress more effectively. It's also a good idea to consult with a healthcare professional or registered dietitian to ensure your goals align with your overall health and well-being.

3.2 Preparing Your Kitchen

The success of the Atkins Diet largely depends on your environment and the availability of appropriate foods. Preparing your kitchen for the diet is a crucial step in ensuring you have the right ingredients and tools at your disposal. Here's how to get your kitchen ready:

- **Purge High-Carb Foods**: Start by clearing your kitchen of high-carb foods such as bread, pasta, rice, sugary snacks, and processed foods. Donate or discard items that don't align with your dietary goals.

- **Stock Up on Low-Carb Staples**: Invest in low-carb staples like lean meats, poultry, fish, eggs, nuts, seeds, low-carb vegetables, and healthy fats (e.g., olive oil, avocado oil). Having these items readily available will make meal preparation easier.

- **Plan Your Meals**: Create a meal plan for the week that includes low-carb recipes and snacks. This will help you stay on track and reduce the temptation to reach for high-carb options when you're hungry.

- **Purchase Keto-Friendly Ingredients**: If you're in the initial phase of the Atkins Diet (Induction Phase), you may need to purchase specific keto-friendly ingredients like coconut oil, MCT oil, and ketone test strips to monitor your ketosis.

- **Food Storage**: Ensure you have appropriate food storage containers to keep prepared meals and leftovers fresh. Organizing your pantry and refrigerator can also help you find what you need easily.

- **Kitchen Equipment**: Check that you have the necessary kitchen equipment, such as pots, pans, and utensils, to prepare low-carb meals effectively.

- **Read Labels**: Familiarize yourself with reading food labels to identify hidden sugars and carbs. Look for items with

minimal added sugars and
carbohydrates.

- **Hydration**: Have an adequate
  supply of water and consider
  incorporating herbal teas or
  flavored sparkling water for
  variety.

- **Snacking Options**: Keep low-
  carb snacks on hand for
  moments when you need a
  quick bite. Options like cheese,
  nuts, and raw vegetables can be
  satisfying choices.

Taking these steps to prepare your kitchen, you'll create an environment that supports your Atkins Diet journey. A well-organized and well-stocked kitchen can help you stay committed to your dietary goals and make the transition to the diet more seamless. Additionally, planning your meals in advance can reduce the likelihood of straying from the diet due to last-minute food decisions.

3.3 Meal Planning and Grocery Shopping

Meal planning and grocery shopping are integral parts of successfully adopting the Atkins Diet. A well-thought-out meal plan ensures that you have nutritious and low-carb options readily available, while efficient grocery shopping helps you stick to your dietary goals and budget. Here's how to navigate meal planning and grocery shopping for the Atkins Diet:

Meal Planning:

1. **Set a Weekly Meal Plan:** Plan your meals for the week ahead,

including breakfast, lunch, dinner, and snacks. Having a structured plan will reduce the likelihood of impulsive, high-carb choices.

2. **Choose Low-Carb Recipes:** Seek out Atkins Diet-friendly recipes that align with your goals and dietary phase. Look for recipes that include lean proteins, healthy fats, and non-starchy vegetables.

3. **Variety**: Incorporate a variety of foods to ensure you receive a broad range of nutrients. Rotate through different protein sources, vegetables, and fats to keep your meals interesting.

4. **Prep Ahead**: Consider preparing some meals or components of meals in

advance to save time during busy days. This might include marinating meats, chopping vegetables, or cooking extra portions for leftovers.

5. **Snack Options**: Include low-carb snacks in your meal plan to help control hunger between meals. Examples include cheese, nuts, Greek yogurt, and raw veggies with dip.

6. **Hydration**: Remember to include water, herbal teas, and other low-carb beverages in your plan to stay adequately hydrated.

Grocery Shopping:

1. **Make a List**: Before heading to the store, create a detailed shopping list based on your meal plan. Stick to the list as

closely as possible to avoid buying unnecessary items.

2. **Read Labels**: When selecting packaged foods, carefully read labels to check for carbohydrate content. Look for items with minimal added sugars and fewer carbohydrates.

3. **Shop the Perimeter**: In most grocery stores, the perimeter is where fresh produce, meat, dairy, and other whole foods are located. Focus your shopping there to avoid processed and high-carb foods found in the aisles.

4. **Stock Up on Staples**: Purchase low-carb staples like lean meats, poultry, fish, eggs, nuts, seeds, non-starchy vegetables, and healthy fats. These items

will form the basis of your Atkins Diet meals.

5. **Consider Frozen and Canned Foods**: Frozen vegetables and canned goods, such as tuna or salmon, can be convenient options and have a longer shelf life.

6. **Fresh Produce**: Select a variety of fresh, low-carb vegetables and some low-sugar fruits if you're in a later phase of the diet.

7. **Dairy**: If you include dairy in your diet, opt for full-fat or low-fat options, as they typically have fewer carbohydrates than fat-free varieties.

8. **Budget Wisely**: Stick to your budget by prioritizing essential

items and avoiding impulse purchases. Buying in bulk can sometimes be cost-effective.

3.4 Tracking Your Progress

Tracking your progress is a crucial aspect of the Atkins Diet journey. It allows you to assess how the diet is working for you and make necessary adjustments. Here's how to effectively track your progress:

1. **Food Diary**: Maintain a food diary or use a mobile app to record everything you eat and drink. Note portion sizes and carbohydrate counts to ensure you're staying within your daily limit.

2. **Weight and Measurements**:
    Regularly weigh yourself and
    take measurements of key areas
    like your waist, hips, and
    thighs. Track these
    measurements over time to
    gauge your progress.

3. **Ketone Testing**: If you're in
    the Induction Phase or
    following a ketogenic version
    of the diet, use ketone test
    strips to monitor your ketosis
    levels.

4. **Blood Sugar Monitoring**: If
    you have diabetes or
    prediabetes, monitor your blood
    sugar levels as recommended
    by your healthcare provider.
    Note any improvements or
    changes.

5. **Energy Levels and Mood**: Pay attention to how you feel. Do you have more energy, better mental clarity, and improved mood? These are potential non-scale victories.

6. **Consult a Dietitian**: Consider consulting with a registered dietitian or nutritionist who specializes in low-carb diets. They can provide personalized guidance, monitor your progress, and make recommendations based on your specific needs and goals.

7. **Set Milestones**: Break your long-term goals into smaller milestones. Celebrate your achievements along the way to stay motivated.

8. **Regular Check-Ins**: Schedule regular check-ins with yourself to review your progress and adjust your meal plan or goals if necessary.

Progress on the Atkins Diet can vary from person to person, and it's essential to be patient and realistic about your expectations. Tracking your progress helps you make informed decisions about your diet and lifestyle, ultimately leading to greater success in achieving your goals.

CHAPTER 4

Induction Phase

The Induction Phase is the initial stage of the Atkins Diet and sets the foundation for the rest of the dietary program. This phase is characterized by strict carbohydrate restriction to induce a state of ketosis, where the body shifts from burning carbohydrates for energy to burning stored fat. In this section, we will delve into the details of the Induction Phase, including its duration, goals, and the types of foods that are allowed.

4.1 Duration and Goals

- **Duration**: The Induction Phase typically lasts for a minimum of two weeks, although some individuals may choose to extend it based on their goals and progress. The duration can vary depending on factors such as the amount of weight to be lost and individual tolerance to low-carb eating.

- **Goals**:

  - **Inducing Ketosis**: The primary goal of the Induction Phase is to induce ketosis. This metabolic state occurs when carbohydrate intake is severely limited, and the body begins to break down stored fat into ketones for energy. Achieving and maintaining ketosis is essential for fat loss during this phase.

- **Rapid Weight Loss**: Many individuals experience rapid weight loss during the Induction Phase due to the initial depletion of glycogen stores and the loss of water weight associated with lower carbohydrate intake.

- **Stabilizing Blood Sugar**: By significantly reducing carbohydrates, the Induction Phase can help stabilize blood sugar levels, making it beneficial for those with insulin resistance or prediabetes.

- **Controlling Appetite**: Ketosis often leads to reduced appetite and cravings, making it easier to control calorie intake.

- **Adapting to Low-Carb Eating**: The Induction Phase helps individuals adapt to a low-carb lifestyle and sets the stage for transitioning to the subsequent phases of the Atkins Diet.

4.2 Allowed Foods

The Induction Phase of the Atkins Diet focuses on very low-carb foods that promote ketosis. Here are some of the key foods that are allowed during this phase:

1. **Proteins**: Lean meats, poultry, fish, and seafood are primary sources of protein. These can include beef, chicken, turkey, pork, salmon, trout, shrimp, and more.

2. **Eggs**: Eggs are an excellent source of protein and healthy fats and are versatile for preparing various dishes.

3. **Fats**: Healthy fats are encouraged during the Induction Phase. This includes fats from sources like olive oil, avocado oil, coconut oil, butter, and animal fats.

4. **Low-Carb Vegetables**: Non-starchy vegetables are a key component of the Induction Phase. Examples include spinach, kale, lettuce, broccoli, cauliflower, zucchini, and asparagus. These vegetables are rich in fiber and nutrients while being low in carbohydrates.

5. **Dairy**: Limited quantities of full-fat dairy products like

cheese and cream are allowed. Be mindful of the carb content in dairy, and choose options with minimal added sugars.

6. **Herbs and Spices**: Use herbs and spices to season your food without adding carbohydrates.

7. **Condiments**: Some condiments like mayonnaise, mustard, and vinegar are permitted in moderation. Be cautious with ketchup and other high-sugar condiments.

8. **Beverages**: Drink plenty of water, herbal teas, and coffee or tea without added sugars. Staying well-hydrated is crucial during this phase.

It's important to note that during the Induction Phase, foods high in carbohydrates are strictly restricted.

This includes grains, bread, pasta, rice, sugary foods, fruits, and starchy vegetables like potatoes and corn.

4.3 Sample Meal Plan

Creating a balanced and satisfying meal plan during the Induction Phase of the Atkins Diet is crucial for success. Here's a sample meal plan to give you an idea of how to structure your meals while staying within the recommended daily carbohydrate limit of around 20-25 grams of net carbs:

Note: Net carbs are calculated by subtracting fiber from total carbohydrates.

Day 1:

Breakfast:

- Scrambled eggs with spinach cooked in butter.

- Side of sliced avocado.

Lunch:

- Grilled chicken breast served over a bed of mixed greens with olive oil and vinegar dressing.

Snack:

- Celery sticks with cream cheese.

Dinner:

- Baked salmon with lemon and dill.

- Steamed broccoli with a pat of butter.

Day 2:

Breakfast:

* Omelette with diced bell peppers, onions, and cheese.

* Sliced tomatoes on the side.

Lunch:

* Tuna salad made with canned tuna, mayo, and chopped pickles. Serve over lettuce leaves.

Snack:

* Handful of mixed nuts (watch portion size to keep carb intake low).

Dinner:

* Grilled shrimp with garlic butter.

* Asparagus spears roasted with olive oil.

Day 3:

Breakfast:

- Full-fat Greek yogurt with a few raspberries (in moderation).

Lunch:

- Beef stir-fry with non-starchy vegetables (bell peppers, broccoli, and snap peas) cooked in olive oil and soy sauce (use sparingly).

Snack:

- Sliced cucumbers with a small portion of hummus.

Dinner:

- Roasted chicken thighs with rosemary and lemon.

- Sautéed spinach with garlic.

4.4 Tips for Success

Successfully navigating the Induction Phase of the Atkins Diet requires commitment and attention to detail. Here are some tips to help you achieve your goals during this phase:

1. **Plan Ahead**: Create a meal plan for the week and prepare your meals in advance when possible. This will help you avoid making high-carb choices due to convenience.

2. **Stay Hydrated**: Drink plenty of water throughout the day to stay hydrated and help flush out waste products as your body adjusts to ketosis.

3. **Monitor Your Carbs**: Keep a food diary or use a mobile app to track your carbohydrate

intake. This will help you stay within your daily limit.

4. **Choose Quality Proteins**: Opt for high-quality, lean sources of protein to keep you feeling full and satisfied.

5. **Incorporate Healthy Fats**: Include healthy fats like avocado, olive oil, and nuts to support your energy needs and overall well-being.

6. **Mind Your Portions**: Pay attention to portion sizes to avoid overeating, even with low-carb foods.

7. **Read Labels**: Carefully read food labels to identify hidden sugars and carbohydrates in packaged products.

8. **Stay Consistent**: Stick to the Induction Phase guidelines consistently to achieve and maintain ketosis.

9. **Monitor Ketosis**: If desired, use ketone test strips to monitor your ketosis levels and confirm that you're in a state of fat burning.

10. **Seek Support**: Consider joining an online community or support group of individuals following the Atkins Diet for motivation and advice.

11. **Consult a Healthcare Professional**: Before starting any diet, especially if you have underlying health conditions or concerns, consult with a healthcare professional or

registered dietitian for guidance and monitoring.

Induction Phase is just the beginning of your Atkins Diet journey. Once you've achieved your initial goals, you can gradually transition to the subsequent phases of the diet, allowing for slightly higher carbohydrate intake while maintaining your progress. Persistence, discipline, and patience are key to success on the Atkins Diet.

CHAPTER 5

Balancing Phase

The Balancing Phase is the second stage of the Atkins Diet, following the Induction Phase. During this phase, you will transition to a higher carbohydrate intake while continuing to lose weight, although at a slower rate compared to the Induction Phase. The Balancing Phase is crucial for determining your individual carbohydrate tolerance and finding a sustainable level of carb consumption. In this section, we will explore how to transition into this phase, adjust your carbohydrate intake, provide a sample meal plan, and offer tips for staying on track.

5.1 Transitioning to the Balancing Phase

Transitioning from the Induction Phase to the Balancing Phase is a gradual process. Here's how to make the transition effectively:

- **Duration**: The Induction Phase typically lasts for a minimum of two weeks, but you can extend it based on your progress and goals. When you decide it's time to move on, you can begin the Balancing Phase.

- **Increase Carbs Gradually**: Slowly introduce additional carbohydrates into your diet. Start with an extra 5-10 grams of net carbs per day for the first week. For example, you might add small portions of berries or nuts.

- **Monitor Your Body**: Pay close attention to how your body responds to the added carbs. Note any changes in weight loss, energy levels, or cravings.

- **Stay in Ketosis (Optional)**: Some individuals choose to maintain a mild state of ketosis even in the Balancing Phase by keeping their carb intake at the lower end of the recommended range. This can vary depending on your personal preferences and goals.

5.2 Adjusting Carbohydrate Intake

During the Balancing Phase, you will gradually adjust your carbohydrate intake to find the right balance for your goals. Here are some general guidelines:

- **Carbohydrate Sources**: Focus on adding more low-carb vegetables, such as cauliflower, broccoli, and leafy greens, as well as small portions of berries, nuts, and seeds.

- **Increase in Increments**: Gradually increase your daily carbohydrate intake by 5-10 grams of net carbs per week, while continuing to monitor your progress. Keep a food diary to track your carb intake accurately.

- **Monitor Weight Loss**: Weight loss may slow down as you increase carb intake, but this is expected. The goal is to find the highest level of carbohydrate

consumption that still allows
for gradual weight loss.

- **Energy Levels**: Assess how
  you feel as you add more carbs.
  If you experience increased
  energy and improved workouts,
  you may be finding your
  carbohydrate sweet spot.

- **Hunger and Cravings**: Watch
  for signs of increased hunger or
  cravings. If you find that
  adding more carbs leads to
  overeating or stalls your
  progress, consider reducing
  your carb intake slightly.

5.3 Sample Meal Plan

Here's a sample meal plan for the
Balancing Phase, which incorporates
a slightly higher level of

carbohydrates than the Induction Phase. Remember to adjust portion sizes and carb sources based on your individual carbohydrate tolerance:

Day 1:

Breakfast:

- Scrambled eggs with sautéed mushrooms and spinach.

- A small serving of mixed berries.

Lunch:

- Grilled chicken salad with mixed greens, cherry tomatoes, and vinaigrette dressing.

Snack:

- Greek yogurt with a drizzle of honey (in moderation).

Dinner:

- Baked cod with lemon and herbs.

- Steamed broccoli with a pat of butter.

- A side salad with avocado and olive oil dressing.

Day 2:

Breakfast:

- Omelette with diced bell peppers, onions, and cheese.

- Sliced tomatoes on the side.

Lunch:

- Tuna salad made with canned tuna, mayo, and chopped pickles. Serve over lettuce leaves.

Snack:

- Sliced cucumber with cream cheese.

Dinner:

- Grilled shrimp skewers with garlic butter.

- Asparagus spears roasted with olive oil.

5.4 Staying on Track

Successfully navigating the Balancing Phase of the Atkins Diet requires diligence and mindful tracking of your carbohydrate intake. Here are some tips to help you stay on track:

1. **Keep Monitoring**: Continue to monitor your carbohydrate intake, weight loss progress, energy levels, and overall well-

being. Adjust your carb consumption as needed.

2. **Portion Control**: Pay attention to portion sizes, especially when adding carbohydrate-rich foods. It's easy to overconsume carbs even with healthy options.

3. **Plan Your Meals**: Maintain a structured meal plan to ensure that you're incorporating the right balance of protein, fats, and carbohydrates in your diet.

4. **Stay Hydrated**: Adequate hydration is essential. Drink plenty of water to support your overall health and well-being.

5. **Regular Exercise**: Incorporate regular physical activity into your routine to enhance weight loss and overall health. Consult

with a fitness professional if needed.

6. **Consult a Dietitian**: If you have specific dietary concerns or goals, consider consulting with a registered dietitian or nutritionist who can provide personalized guidance and meal planning assistance.

7. **Mindful Eating**: Practice mindful eating by paying attention to hunger and fullness cues. Avoid emotional eating or eating out of habit.

8. **Flexibility**: Be flexible with your approach. The Balancing Phase is about finding what works best for you. Adjustments may be necessary based on your individual

responses to different carb levels.

9. **Seek Support**: Consider joining a support group or online community of individuals following the Atkins Diet for motivation and advice.

10. **Celebrate Milestones**: Celebrate your achievements and milestones along the way to stay motivated and focused on your long-term goals.

The Balancing Phase is a crucial step in your Atkins Diet journey. It allows you to fine-tune your carbohydrate intake, continue your weight loss progress, and find a sustainable eating pattern that you can maintain over the long term.

CHAPTER 6

Pre-Maintenance Phase

The Pre-Maintenance Phase is the third stage of the Atkins Diet, following the Induction Phase and the Balancing Phase. During this phase, you'll prepare your body for long-term maintenance and further refine your carbohydrate intake to find the optimal level for your individual needs. In this section, we will explore how to transition into the Pre-Maintenance Phase, gradually reintroduce carbohydrates, monitor your progress, and provide a sample meal plan.

6.1 Preparing for Maintenance

Transitioning from the Balancing Phase to the Pre-Maintenance Phase involves preparing both mentally and practically for a more flexible approach to carbohydrate intake:

- **Mindset**: Embrace the idea of a more balanced and sustainable approach to eating. The Pre-Maintenance Phase is about finding your individual carbohydrate tolerance while maintaining your progress.

- **Set Goals**: Define your goals for the Pre-Maintenance Phase. Are you primarily focused on reaching your target weight, managing blood sugar, or simply maintaining your current weight?

- **Consult a Professional**:
Consider consulting with a
registered dietitian or
healthcare professional to
create a plan tailored to your
specific goals and needs.

6.2 Gradually Reintroducing Carbs

During the Pre-Maintenance Phase,
you'll gradually reintroduce
carbohydrates into your diet while
monitoring your body's response.
Here are some guidelines:

- **Incremental Increases**:
Increase your daily
carbohydrate intake by 10-20
grams of net carbs per week,
while closely monitoring your
progress.

- **Choose Quality Carbs**:
  Prioritize complex
  carbohydrates from whole
  foods, such as whole grains,
  legumes, and additional fruits
  and vegetables.

- **Monitor Your Body**: Pay
  attention to how your body
  responds to the increased
  carbohydrate intake. Note
  changes in weight, energy
  levels, and any signs of
  cravings or hunger.

- **Find Your Balance**: The goal
  is to find the maximum level of
  carbohydrate consumption that
  allows you to maintain your
  weight without gaining it back.
  This level will vary from
  person to person.

6.3 Monitoring Your Progress

As you transition through the Pre-Maintenance Phase, it's essential to monitor your progress and make adjustments as needed. Here's how to do it effectively:

- **Regular Weigh-Ins**: Continue weighing yourself regularly and taking measurements to track your progress.

- **Assess Energy Levels**: Pay attention to your energy levels and overall well-being. Ensure that you have enough energy for your daily activities and exercise.

- **Hunger and Cravings**: Monitor your appetite and cravings. Adjust your

carbohydrate intake if you
notice increased hunger or
uncontrollable cravings.

- **Blood Sugar**: If you have
diabetes or prediabetes,
continue to monitor your blood
sugar levels as recommended
by your healthcare provider.

- **Consult a Dietitian**: If you
have specific dietary concerns
or goals, consult with a
registered dietitian or
nutritionist for ongoing support
and guidance.

6.4 Sample Meal Plan

Here's a sample meal plan for the Pre-
Maintenance Phase, which includes a
moderate level of carbohydrates.
Adjust portion sizes and carb sources

based on your individual carbohydrate tolerance and goals:

Day 1:

Breakfast:

- Greek yogurt with mixed berries and a drizzle of honey (in moderation).

Lunch:

- Grilled chicken breast with quinoa and a side of roasted mixed vegetables.

Snack:

- Sliced cucumbers with hummus.

Dinner:

- Baked salmon with a quinoa and spinach salad dressed with vinaigrette.

Day 2:

Breakfast:

- Oatmeal topped with sliced bananas and chopped nuts.

Lunch:

- Lentil and vegetable soup with a side of whole-grain crackers.

Snack:

- Handful of mixed nuts (portion size depends on individual tolerance).

Dinner:

- Grilled tofu with a side of brown rice and steamed broccoli.

Day 3:

Breakfast:

- Scrambled eggs with diced tomatoes and a slice of whole-grain toast.

Lunch:

- Spinach and feta-stuffed chicken breast with quinoa salad.

Snack:

- Sliced bell peppers with guacamole.

Dinner:

- Grilled shrimp with a side of whole-wheat pasta and garlic sautéed spinach.

The Pre-Maintenance Phase of the Atkins Diet is a critical step in your journey toward long-term weight management and overall health. By gradually reintroducing carbohydrates while monitoring your body's response, you can find the right balance that allows you to maintain your desired weight and well-being. Remember that individual carbohydrate tolerance varies, so it's essential to customize your approach based on your specific goals and needs. Consulting with a healthcare professional or dietitian can provide valuable guidance during this phase.

CHAPTER 7

Maintenance Phase

The Maintenance Phase is the final stage of the Atkins Diet, following the Induction Phase, Balancing Phase, and Pre-Maintenance Phase. During this phase, you will have reached your target weight or health goals and are focused on maintaining your progress over the long term. In this section, we will explore the key aspects of the Maintenance Phase, including its emphasis on long-term sustainability and finding your individual carbohydrate tolerance.

7.1 Long-Term Sustainability

The Maintenance Phase of the Atkins Diet is all about achieving long-term sustainability. Here's what you need to consider:

- **Lifestyle Change**: Embrace the Maintenance Phase as a permanent lifestyle change rather than a temporary diet. This phase is designed to help you maintain your weight, health improvements, and overall well-being for years to come.

- **Balanced Approach**: Maintain a balanced and flexible approach to your diet. While the previous phases involved strict carbohydrate restrictions, the Maintenance Phase allows for more flexibility in your food choices.

- **Individualized Plan**: Your carbohydrate tolerance is unique, so your maintenance plan should be tailored to your needs. This means finding the right balance of carbohydrates, fats, and protein that allows you to maintain your desired weight and health.

- **Mindful Eating**: Continue practicing mindful eating habits, such as paying attention to portion sizes and recognizing hunger and fullness cues. Avoid emotional eating or overindulgence.

- **Regular Exercise**: Incorporate regular physical activity into your routine. Exercise is an essential component of long-term weight maintenance and overall health.

- **Monitor Progress**: Periodically assess your progress and make adjustments as needed. Keep an eye on your weight, energy levels, and overall well-being.

- **Consult a Dietitian**: Consider consulting with a registered dietitian or nutritionist who specializes in weight maintenance and long-term health. They can provide personalized guidance and support.

7.2 Finding Your Carb Tolerance

Finding your individual carbohydrate tolerance is a crucial aspect of the Maintenance Phase. It involves determining the maximum level of carbohydrate consumption that allows you to maintain your desired weight and health. Here's how to approach this:

- **Gradual Increases**: Continue gradually increasing your daily carbohydrate intake, monitoring your body's response each step of the way. Increase by 10-20 grams of net carbs per week.

- **Keep Track**: Maintain a food diary to record your daily carbohydrate intake, along with other key information like weight, energy levels, and any signs of cravings or hunger.

- **Monitor Weight**: Regularly weigh yourself and take measurements to ensure that your weight remains stable. This will help you identify the right balance of carbs for maintenance.

- **Energy and Well-Being**: Pay attention to your energy levels and overall well-being. Your carbohydrate tolerance should allow you to feel energized and satisfied without significant fluctuations in weight.

- **Hunger and Cravings**: If you experience increased hunger or cravings as you add more carbs, it may be a sign that you're approaching your upper limit of

carbohydrate tolerance.
Consider reducing your carb
intake slightly.

- **Consult a Dietitian**: A
  registered dietitian or
  nutritionist can help you fine-
  tune your maintenance plan
  based on your unique needs and
  goals. They can also provide
  guidance on portion sizes and
  meal planning.

- **Be Patient**: Finding your
  carbohydrate tolerance may
  take time and experimentation.
  Be patient and willing to make
  adjustments as needed to
  maintain your desired results.

The Maintenance Phase is a
continuation of your journey toward
better health and long-term weight
management. It's an opportunity to

enjoy a variety of foods in moderation while maintaining the progress you've achieved. By focusing on sustainability and finding your carbohydrate tolerance, you can make the Maintenance Phase a successful and enjoyable part of your healthy lifestyle.

7.3 Meal Planning for Maintenance

Meal planning remains essential during the Maintenance Phase of the Atkins Diet. While you have more flexibility with your carbohydrate intake, it's crucial to continue making nutritious choices to support your long-term health and weight maintenance. Here's how to approach meal planning during this phase:

1. **Balanced Macronutrients**:
   Plan meals that include a
   balance of carbohydrates,
   healthy fats, and protein. This
   balance can help you feel
   satisfied and provide sustained
   energy throughout the day.

2. **Quality Carbohydrates**:
   Prioritize complex
   carbohydrates from whole
   foods like whole grains,
   legumes, and an array of
   colorful vegetables and fruits.
   These foods are rich in fiber,
   vitamins, and minerals.

3. **Protein**: Continue to
   incorporate lean sources of
   protein like poultry, fish, lean
   meats, tofu, and plant-based
   protein sources. Protein can
   help you maintain muscle mass
   and feel full.

4. **Healthy Fats**: Include sources
    of healthy fats such as
    avocados, nuts, seeds, olive oil,
    and fatty fish like salmon.
    These fats are heart-healthy and
    can support overall well-being.

5. **Portion Control**: Be mindful
    of portion sizes. Even during
    maintenance, overeating can
    lead to weight gain. Pay
    attention to hunger and fullness
    cues.

6. **Variety**: Enjoy a variety of
    foods to ensure you receive a
    broad range of nutrients. Rotate
    through different fruits,
    vegetables, proteins, and grains
    to keep your meals interesting.

7. **Hydration**: Continue to drink
    plenty of water throughout the
    day. Staying hydrated is

essential for overall health and can help control hunger.

8. **Snacking**: Be mindful of snacking. While it's okay to enjoy healthy snacks in moderation, grazing throughout the day can lead to excess calorie intake. Focus on balanced, satisfying meals.

9. **Treats in Moderation**: It's okay to indulge in occasional treats or higher-carb foods. Just be sure to do so in moderation and balance them with other nutritious choices.

10. **Regular Exercise**: Continue with regular physical activity. Exercise is a valuable tool for maintaining weight and overall well-being.

11. **Monitoring**: Periodically revisit your meal plan and assess your progress. Make adjustments as needed to maintain your desired weight and health.

7.4 Avoiding Common Pitfalls

As you navigate the Maintenance Phase, it's important to be aware of common pitfalls that could hinder your progress. Here are some pitfalls to avoid:

1. **Overindulging in Carbs**: Be mindful not to overindulge in carbohydrates, especially refined or sugary options. Overconsumption can lead to

weight gain and blood sugar spikes.

2. **Skipping Meals**: Skipping meals can lead to overeating later in the day. Maintain regular meal times and include a balance of nutrients.

3. **Ignoring Portion Sizes**: Even during maintenance, portion control matters. Be aware of portion sizes to prevent unintentional overeating.

4. **Lack of Physical Activity**: Maintaining regular physical activity is crucial for long-term weight maintenance and overall health. Avoid becoming sedentary.

5. **Mindless Eating**: Avoid eating out of habit or boredom. Pay attention to hunger and fullness

cues to prevent unnecessary snacking.

6. **Not Monitoring Progress**: Periodically assess your weight, energy levels, and overall well-being. Failure to monitor your progress can lead to unwanted weight gain.

7. **Stress and Emotional Eating**: Be mindful of emotional eating and find healthy ways to manage stress and emotions without turning to food.

8. **Ignoring Your Individual Needs**: Everyone's carbohydrate tolerance is unique. Don't compare your maintenance plan to others. Focus on what works best for you.

9. **Not Seeking Support**: If you encounter challenges or need guidance, consider seeking support from a registered dietitian, nutritionist, or a support group for accountability and advice.

10. **Becoming Complacent**: Avoid becoming complacent with your healthy habits. Maintenance is an ongoing process that requires continued commitment.

By being aware of these common pitfalls and proactively addressing them, you can maintain your progress during the Maintenance Phase and enjoy a sustainable, healthy lifestyle for years to come. Remember that the journey toward better health and well-being is a lifelong one, and the

Maintenance Phase is a significant milestone in that journey.

CHAPTER 8

Tips and Tricks

Successfully following the Atkins Diet and achieving your health and weight goals can be made easier with some helpful tips and tricks. In this section, we'll explore how to dine out on the Atkins Diet, handle cravings, incorporate exercise, and stay motivated throughout your journey.

8.1 Dining Out on the Atkins Diet

Dining out while following the Atkins Diet is entirely possible with a bit of planning and awareness. Here's how to navigate restaurant meals:

- **Check the Menu in Advance**: Before going to a restaurant, review the menu online if possible. Look for low-carb options and plan your order accordingly.

- **Choose Protein-Rich Dishes**: Opt for dishes that feature lean proteins like grilled chicken, fish, or steak. Avoid dishes with heavy breading or high-carb sauces.

- **Ask for Modifications**: Don't hesitate to ask the server for modifications to your meal. For example, request vegetables instead of potatoes or a salad instead of bread.

- **Skip the Bread Basket**: Politely decline the bread basket when it's brought to the table to avoid unnecessary carb consumption.

- **Be Mindful of Sauces and Dressings**: Many sauces and dressings can be high in hidden sugars and carbs. Ask for dressings on the side and inquire about sauce ingredients.

- **Share Desserts**: If you're dining with others, consider sharing a dessert rather than indulging in one on your own.

- **Portion Control**: Pay attention to portion sizes, as restaurant portions tend to be larger than necessary. Consider asking for a to-go box to save part of your meal for later.

- **Choose Grilled or Steamed**: Look for menu items that are

grilled, steamed, or roasted
rather than fried or breaded.

- **Drink Water**: Opt for water,
  sparkling water, or
  unsweetened iced tea as your
  beverage to avoid empty
  calories from sugary drinks.

8.2 Handling Cravings

Dealing with cravings is a common
challenge when following any diet.
Here are some strategies for handling
cravings on the Atkins Diet:

- **Identify Triggers**: Pay
  attention to what triggers your
  cravings. Is it stress, boredom,
  or a particular food?
  Understanding your triggers
  can help you address them
  more effectively.

- **Plan Ahead**: Have low-carb snacks or alternatives on hand for when cravings strike. This could include cheese, nuts, or sugar-free treats.

- **Stay Hydrated**: Sometimes thirst can be mistaken for hunger. Drink a glass of water before reaching for a snack to see if your craving subsides.

- **Practice Mindful Eating**: When you do indulge in a treat, savor it mindfully. Eat slowly, savor the flavors, and pay attention to your body's fullness cues.

- **Distract Yourself**: Engage in a distracting activity when cravings hit, such as going for a walk, reading a book, or talking to a friend.

- **Incorporate Variety**: Include a variety of foods in your diet to help prevent food boredom and cravings for specific items.

- **Carb Substitutes**: Explore low-carb substitutes for your favorite high-carb foods. For example, cauliflower can be used to make a pizza crust or mashed potato alternative.

- **Stay Committed to Your Goals**: Remind yourself of the reasons you started the Atkins Diet and the progress you've made. This can help you stay focused on your goals.

8.3 Incorporating Exercise

Exercise is a valuable complement to the Atkins Diet for overall health and weight management. Here's how to incorporate exercise effectively:

- **Choose Activities You Enjoy**: Find physical activities that you genuinely enjoy, whether it's walking, swimming, dancing, or hiking. This makes it more likely that you'll stick with them.

- **Set Realistic Goals**: Set achievable fitness goals that align with your abilities and schedule. Gradually increase the intensity and duration of your workouts over time.

- **Create a Routine**: Establish a regular exercise routine that fits into your daily life. Consistency is key for long-term success.

- **Mix It Up**: Include a variety of activities to prevent boredom and work different muscle groups. This also helps prevent plateaus in your fitness progress.

- **Include Strength Training**: Strength training exercises can help build muscle, boost metabolism, and improve overall body composition.

- **Stay Hydrated**: Drink water before, during, and after your workouts to stay properly hydrated.

- **Listen to Your Body**: Pay attention to how your body responds to exercise. If you experience pain or discomfort, consult with a healthcare professional.

- **Warm Up and Cool Down**: Always start with a warm-up and finish with a cool-down to prevent injuries.

- **Track Your Progress**: Keep a fitness journal to track your workouts and progress. Celebrate your achievements along the way.

8.4 Staying Motivated

Staying motivated throughout your Atkins Diet journey is essential for success. Here are some strategies to help you stay motivated:

- **Set Clear Goals**: Define your short-term and long-term goals, and regularly revisit them to stay focused.

- **Celebrate Achievements**: Acknowledge and celebrate your achievements, no matter how small. This can boost your confidence and motivation.

- **Find a Support System**: Share your goals with friends, family, or a support group. Having a support system can provide encouragement and accountability.

- **Visualize Success**: Imagine yourself reaching your goals and enjoying the benefits of a healthier lifestyle. Visualization can be a powerful motivator.

- **Track Your Progress**: Keep a record of your achievements, whether it's weight loss, improved energy levels, or other positive changes.

- **Reward Yourself**: Treat yourself to non-food rewards when you reach milestones. This can provide extra motivation.

- **Stay Informed**: Continue learning about nutrition, health, and fitness to stay engaged and informed about your journey.

- **Stay Positive**: Cultivate a positive mindset. Focus on what you can do rather than what you can't. Avoid self-criticism and be kind to yourself.

- **Adapt and Adjust**: Be open to making adjustments to your plan as needed. If something isn't working, consider trying a new approach.

- **Visual Reminders**: Use visual reminders of your goals, such as inspirational quotes or images, as motivation.

Motivation can ebb and flow, but maintaining a positive and determined mindset will help you overcome challenges and continue making progress on the Atkins Diet. Your journey is a marathon, not a sprint, and the key is to stay committed to your health and well-being over the long term.